ALLERGY AWARENESS STATE

"According to FoodAllergy.org, 85 million Americans are living with life-threatening food allergies or intolerances, and every 3 minutes, a food allergy reaction sends someone to the emergency room.*

Awareness of food allergies is not just an issue of personal health but also a communal responsibility. So it's a great thing to talk to kids about early.

We thought it would be fun to make a Christmas kid's book where one of the purposes is to teach this important concept about health. We chose food allergies because they can be especially dangerous; you never know unless you ask if someone has a food allergy. Who knows, maybe even Santa Claus has one (good thing it's not to cookies!)

By spreading knowledge and fostering empathy from an early age, we can help future generations grow up with a greater understanding of things like allergies, leading to a more compassionate and safe society for everyone.

For more information visit
https://www.fda.gov/food/food-labeling-nutrition/food-allergies"

Nurse Blake

*https://www.foodallergy.org/resources/facts-and-statistics

Dedicated to those who spend their time (and Christmas) caring for others. Thank you for all your support.

- Nurse Blake

First Edition, 2023
ISBN (Hardback): 978-1-961462-02-1
ISBN (Paperback): 978-1-961462-03-8
ISBN (eBook): 978-1-961462-04-5

"Nurse Blake's Santa Sent to the E.R."
© 2023 by Nurse Blake
All Rights Reserved
Created in collaboration with Timmy Bauer

No part of this book may be reproduced, stored in a retrieval system, or transmitted by any means without the written permission of the author and publisher.

Produced and Published by Dinosaur House,
a children's book production company.

Dinosaur House
DinosaurHouse.com

Published in the United States of America
1 2 3 4 5 6 7 8 9 10

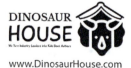

www.DinosaurHouse.com   www.NurseBlake.com

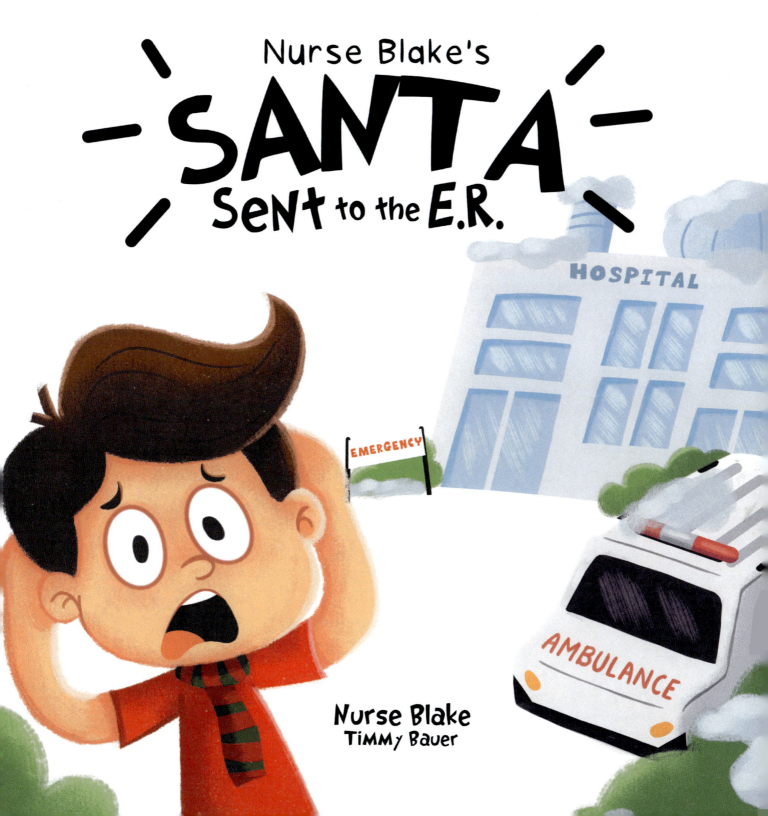

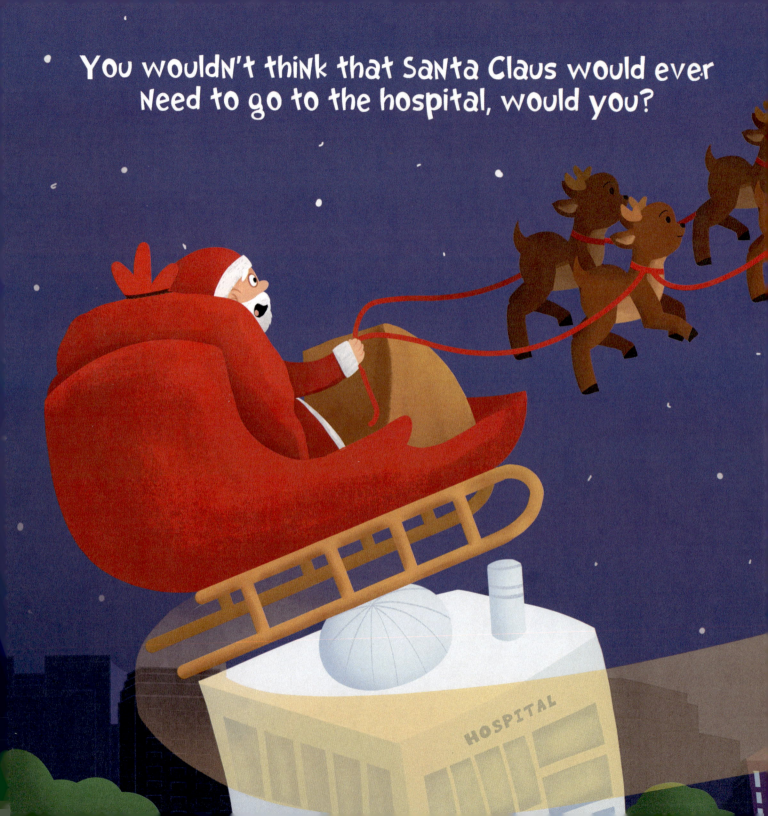
You wouldn't think that Santa Claus would ever need to go to the hospital, would you?

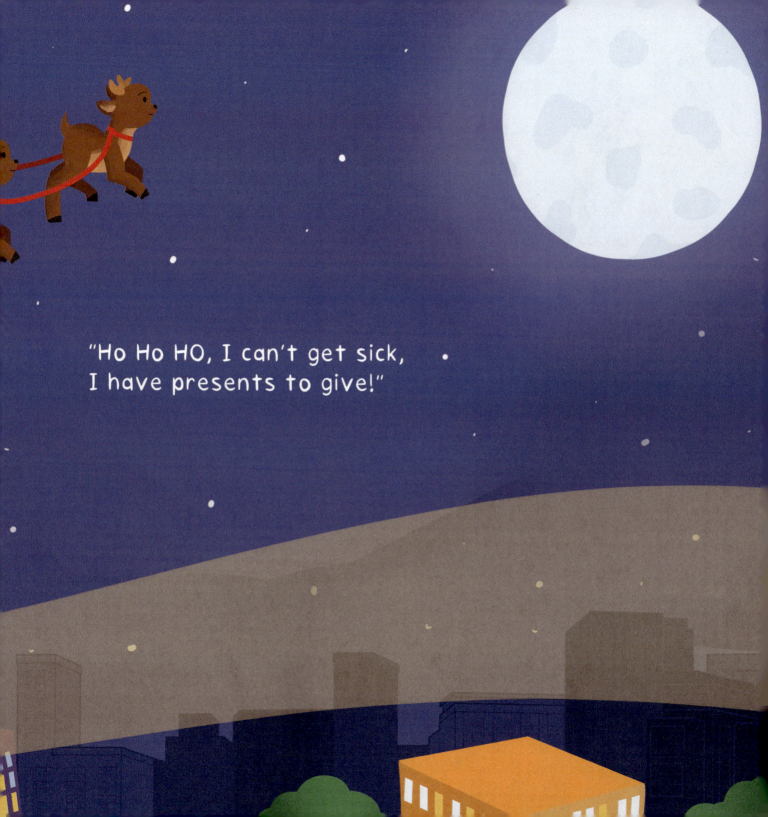

"Ho Ho HO, I can't get sick,
I have presents to give!"

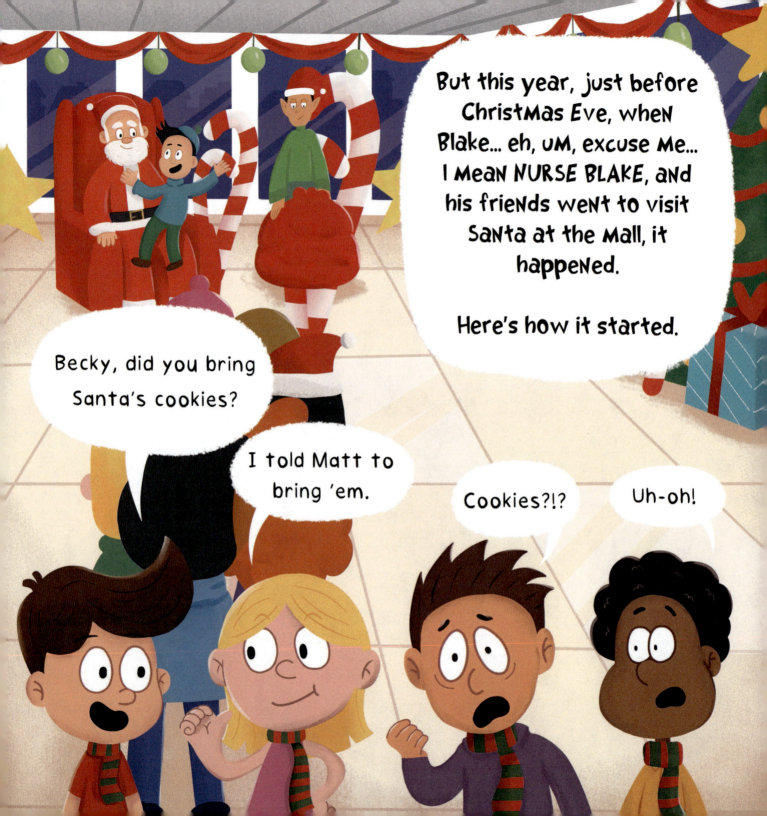

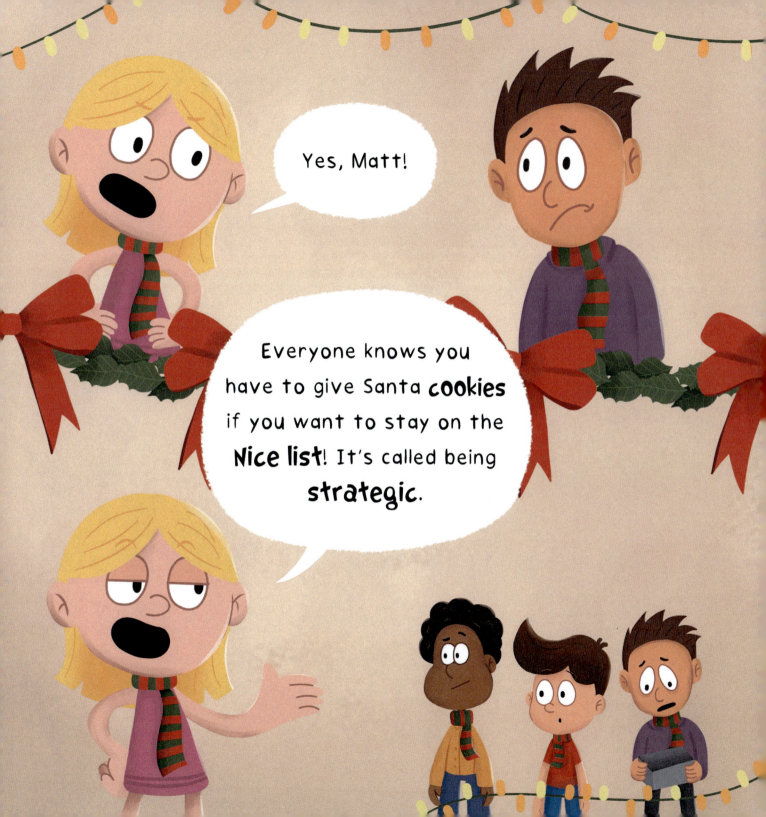

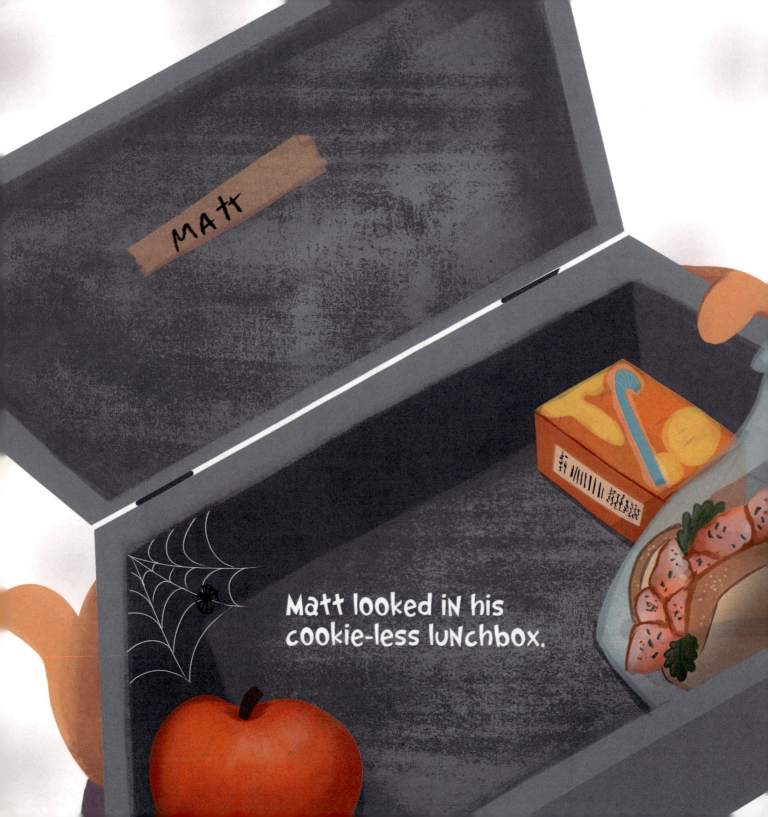

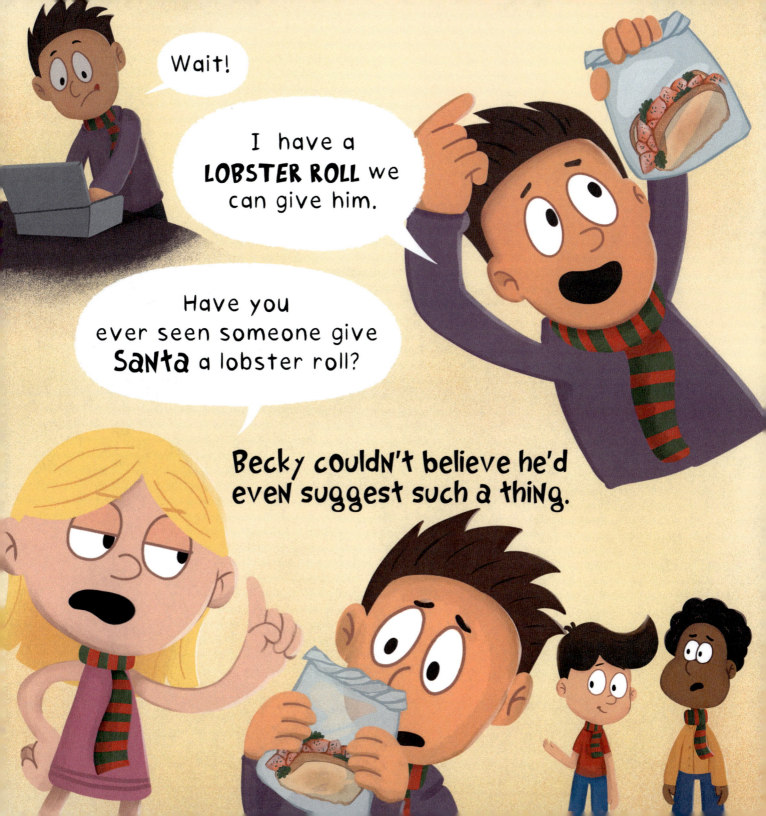

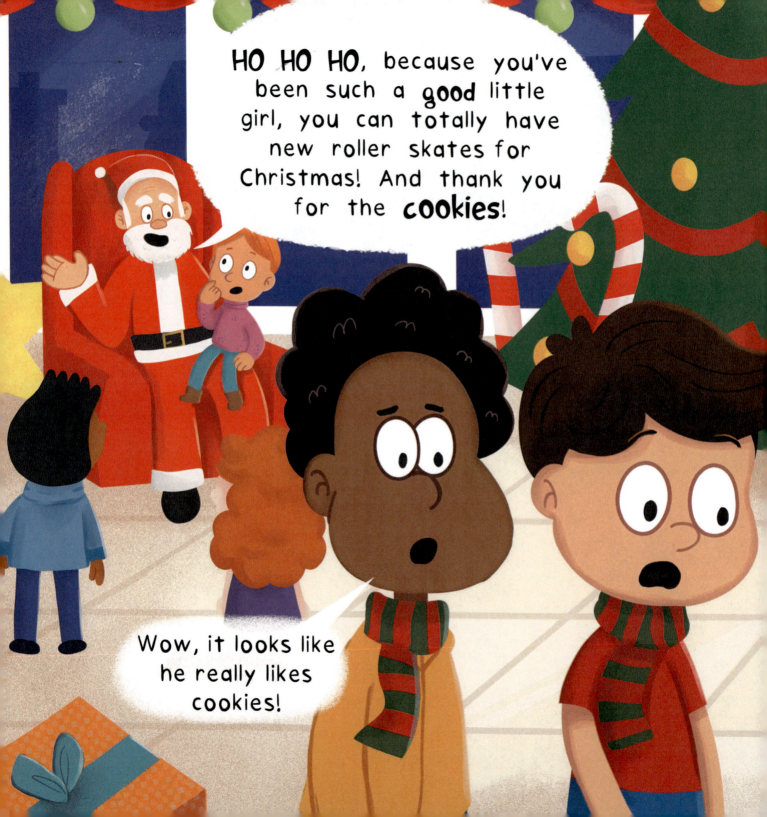

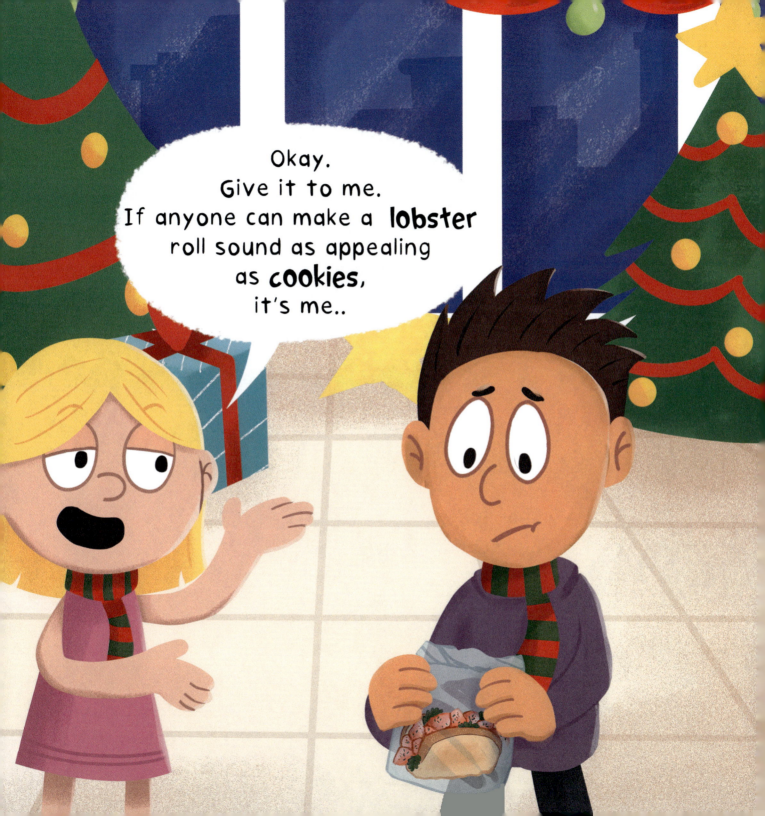

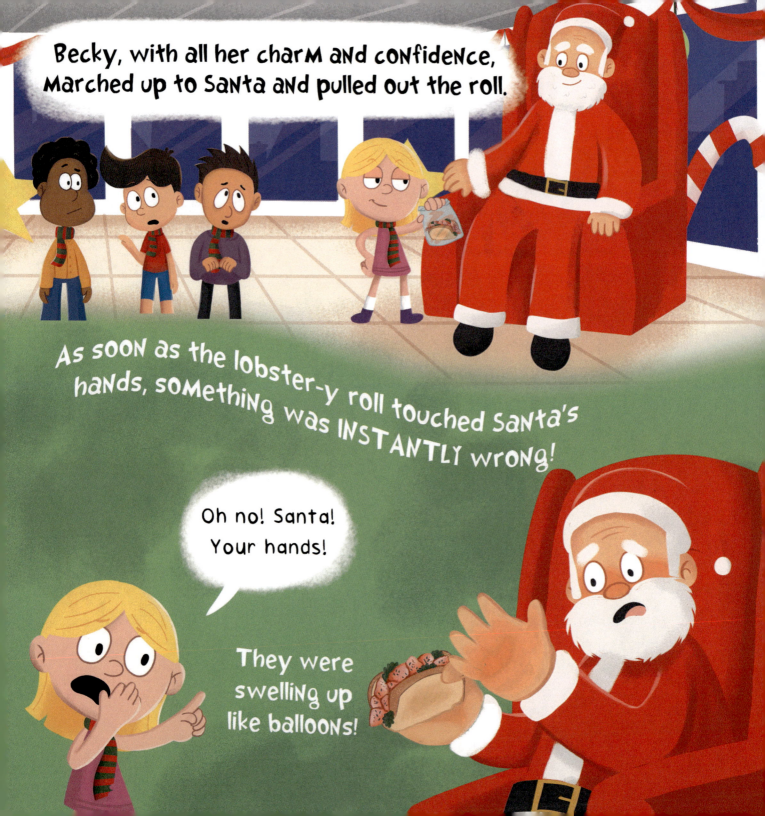

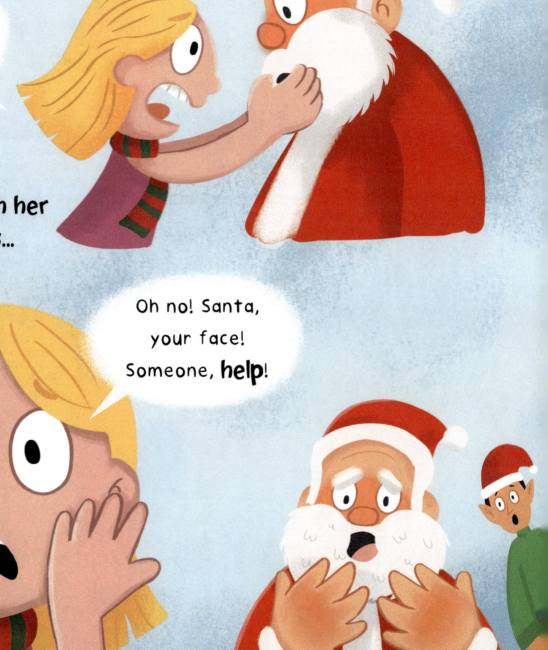

"What's happening to you, Santa?!?"

Becky grabbed Santa's face with her lobster-y fingers... Not a good idea!

"Oh no! Santa, your face! Someone, **help**!"

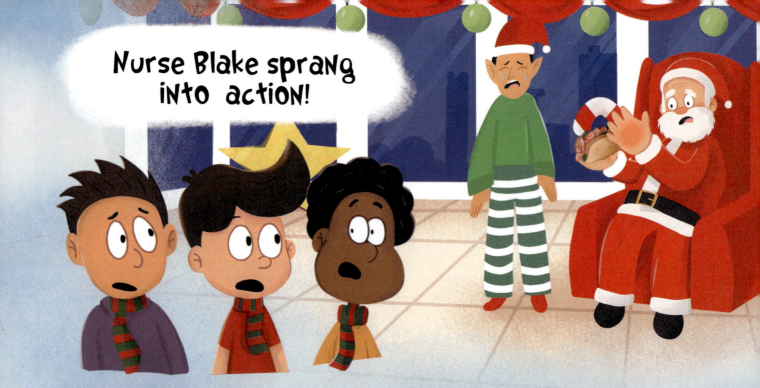

"Nurse Blake sprang into action!"

He remembered all the nursing steps. Do you?

Step 1: (Make sure the scene is safe!)

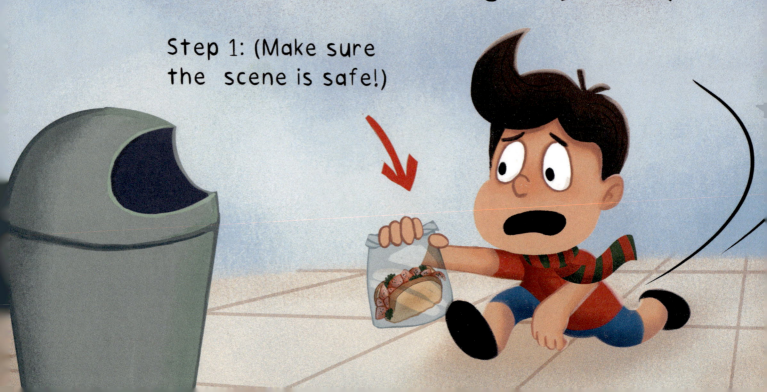

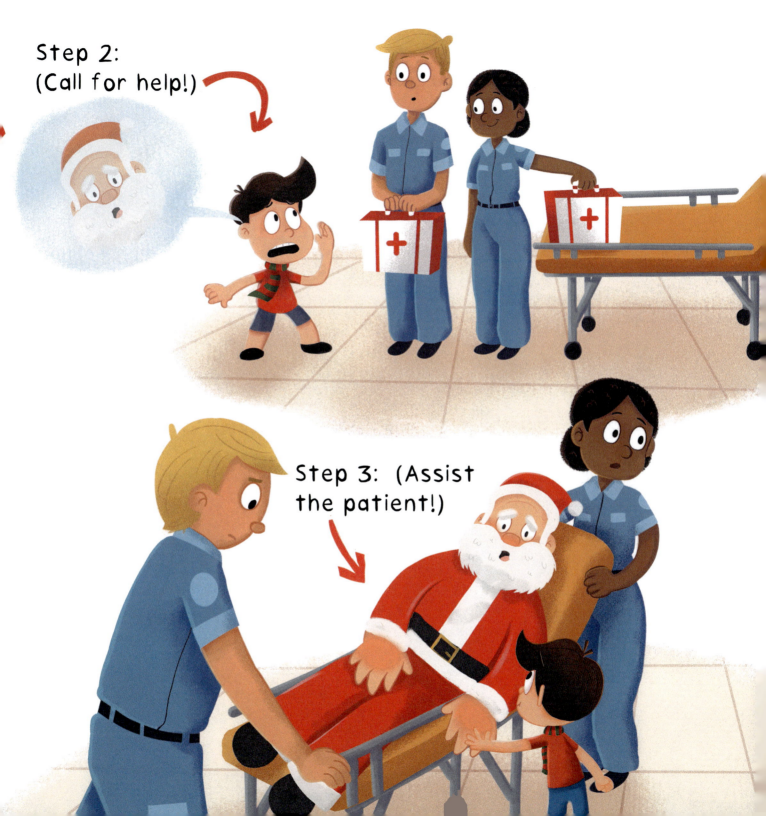

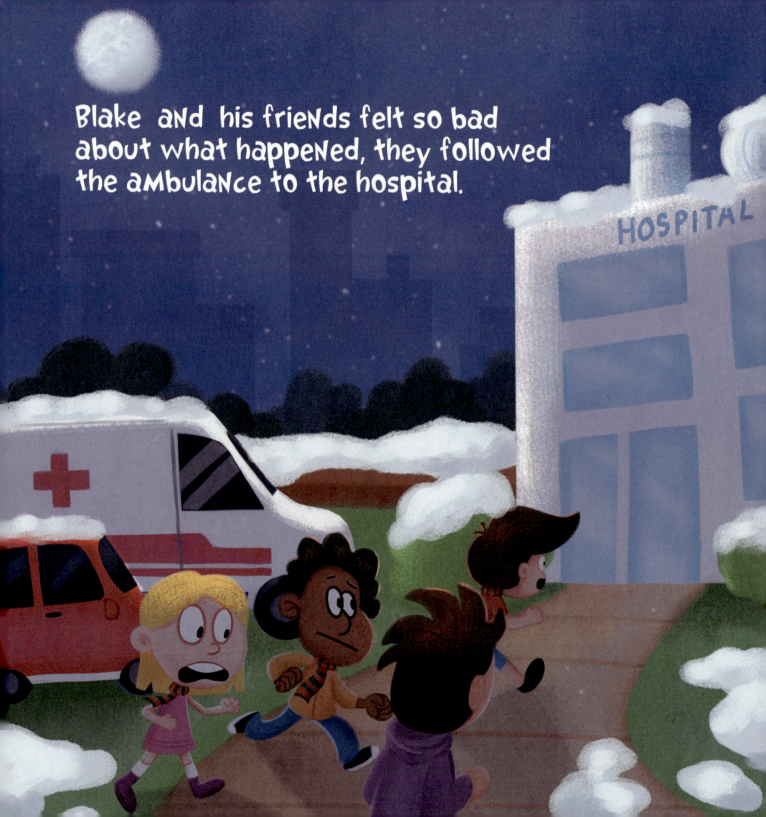
Blake and his friends felt so bad about what happened, they followed the ambulance to the hospital.

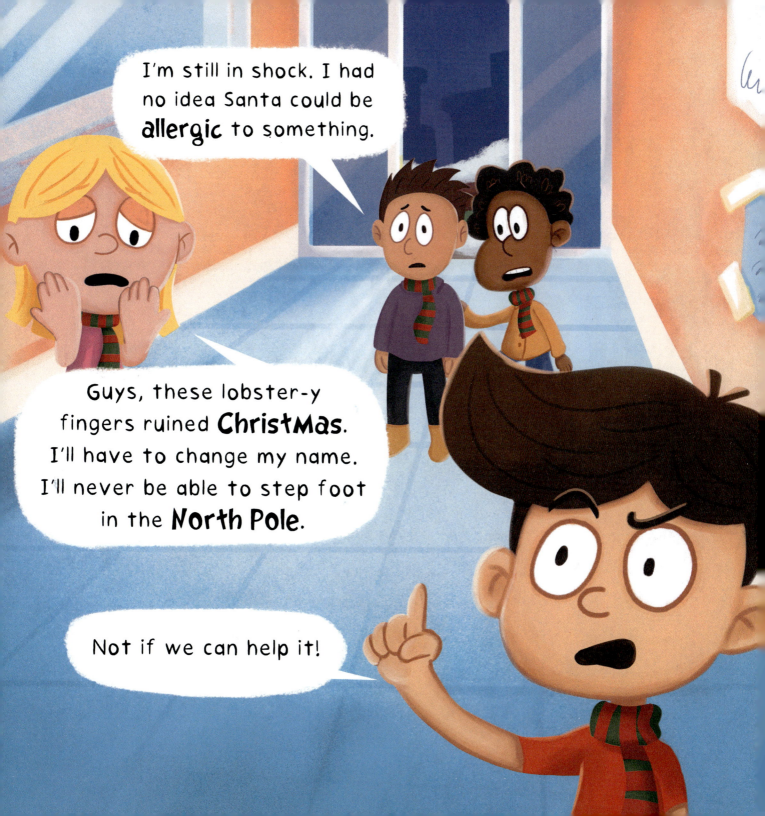

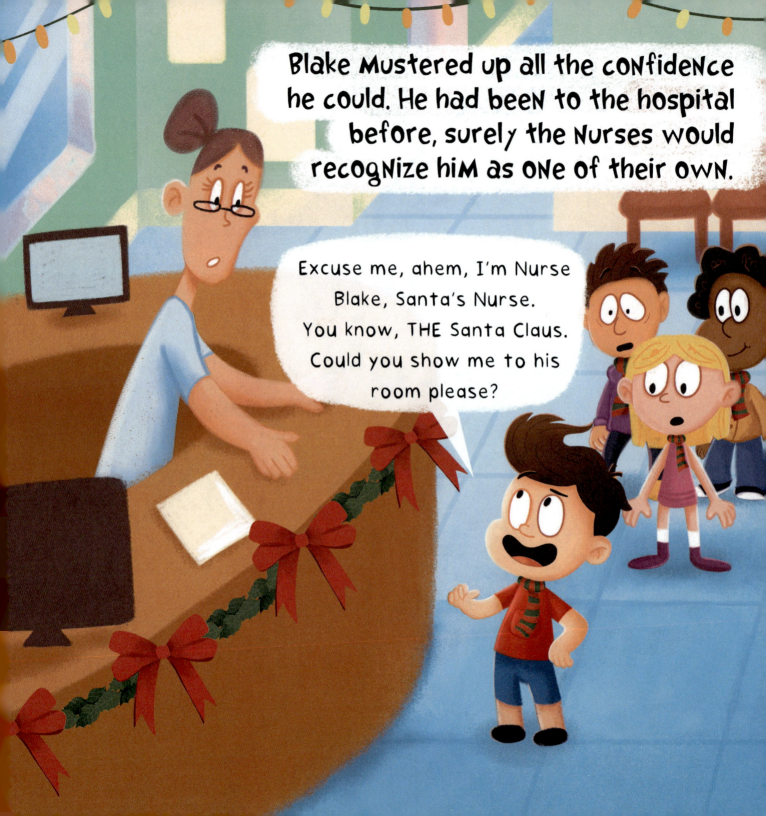

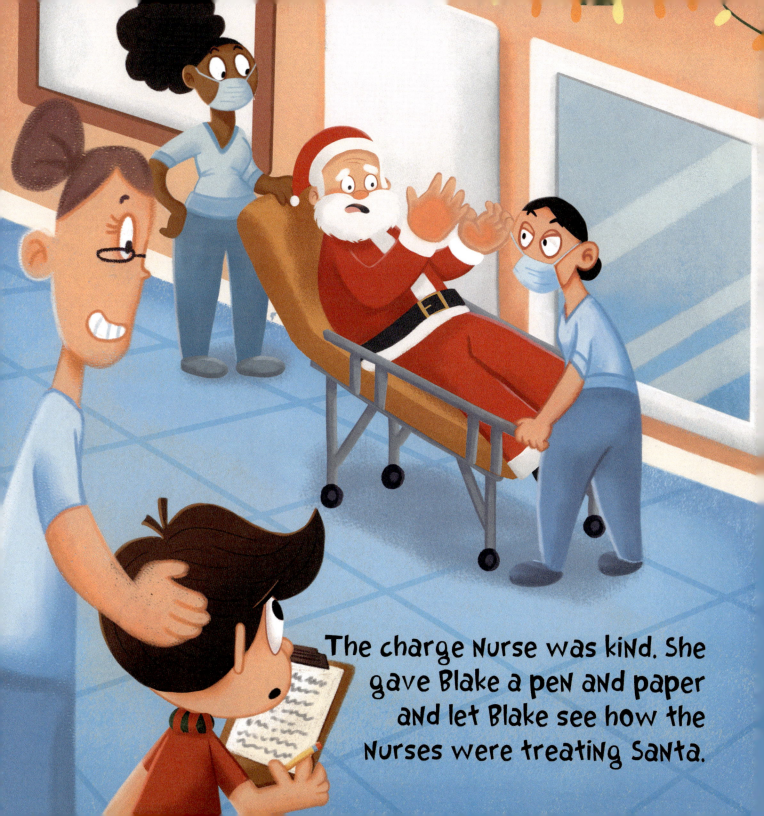

The charge nurse was kind. She gave Blake a pen and paper and let Blake see how the nurses were treating Santa.

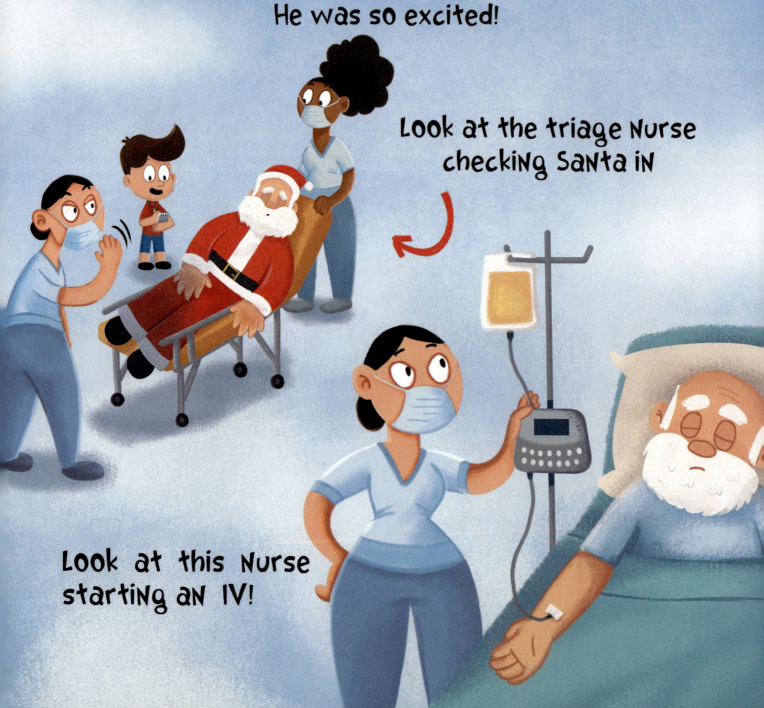

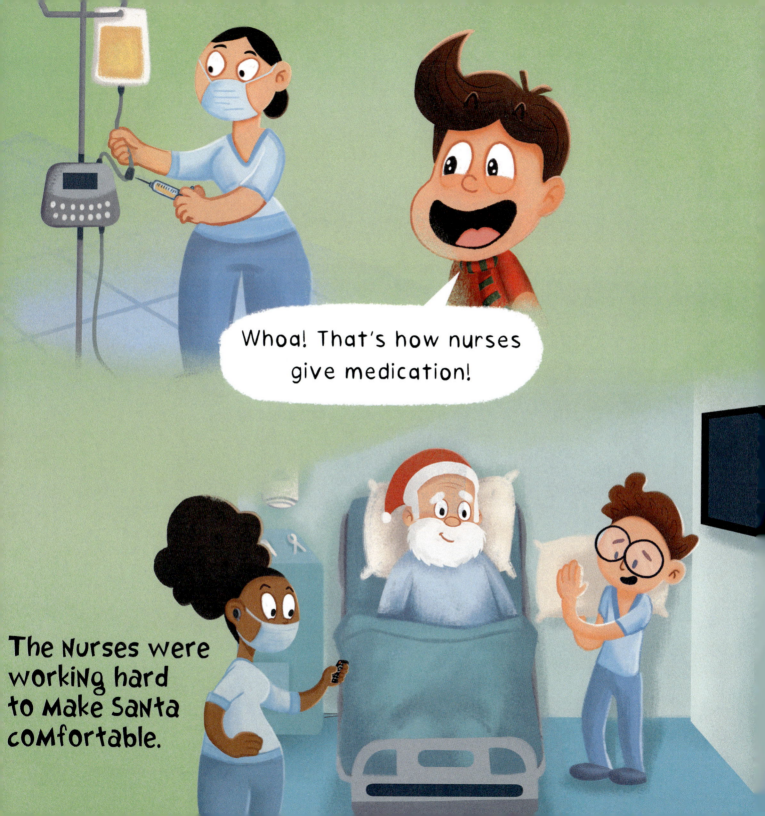

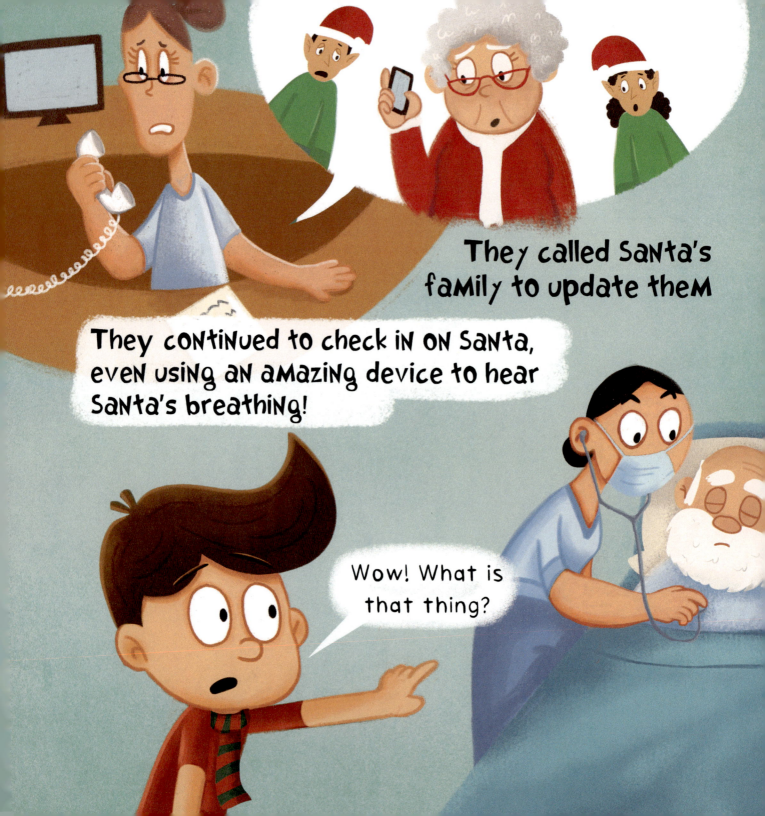

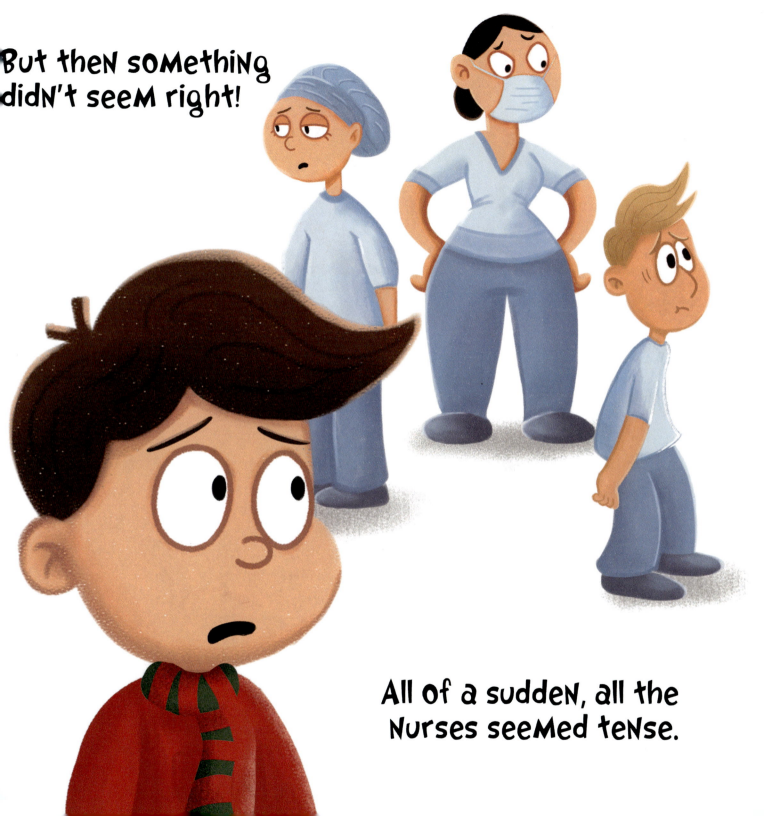

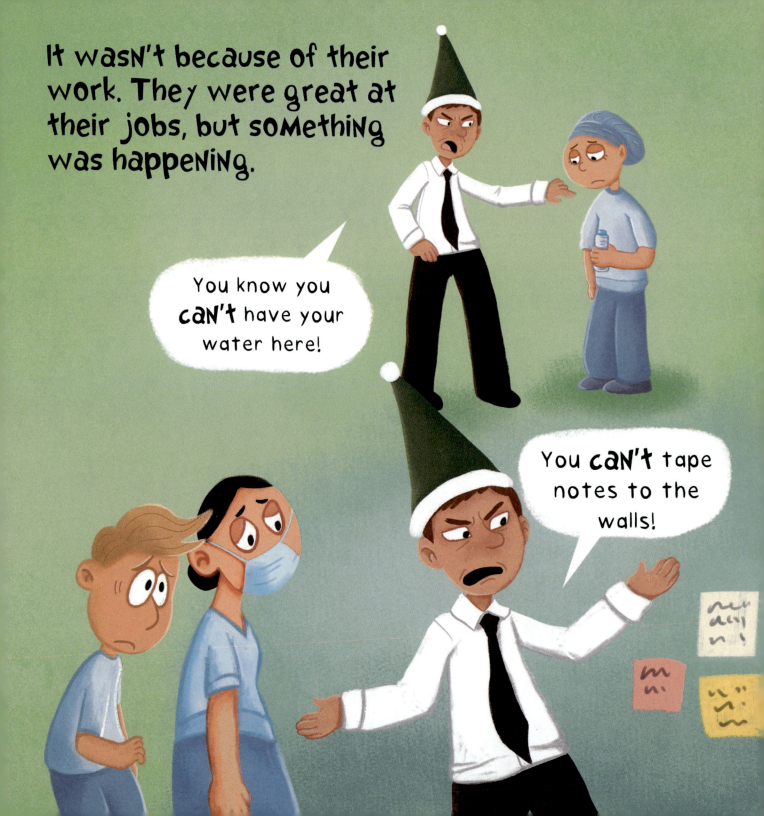

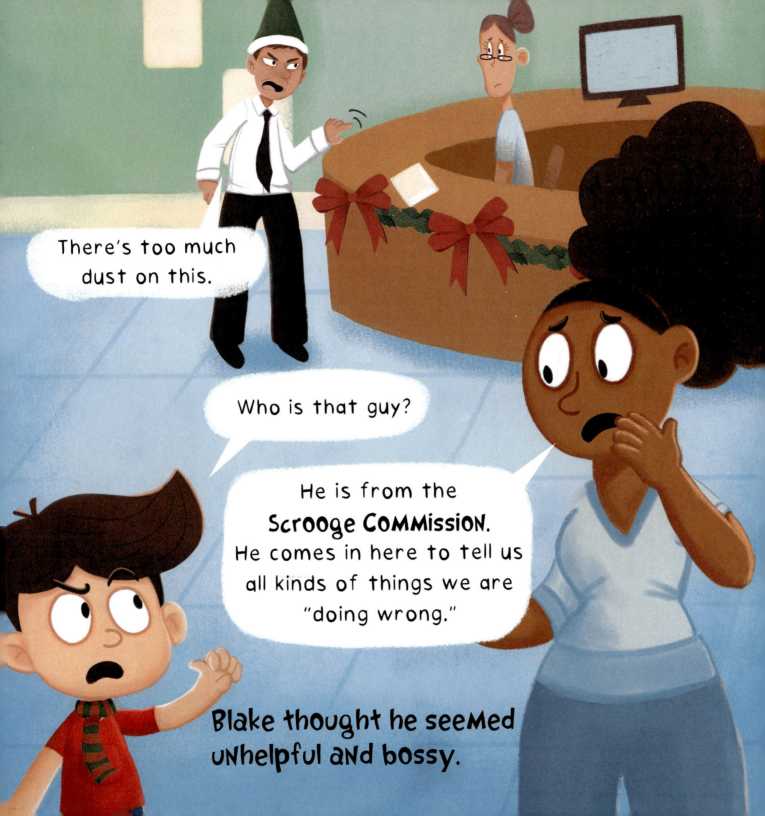

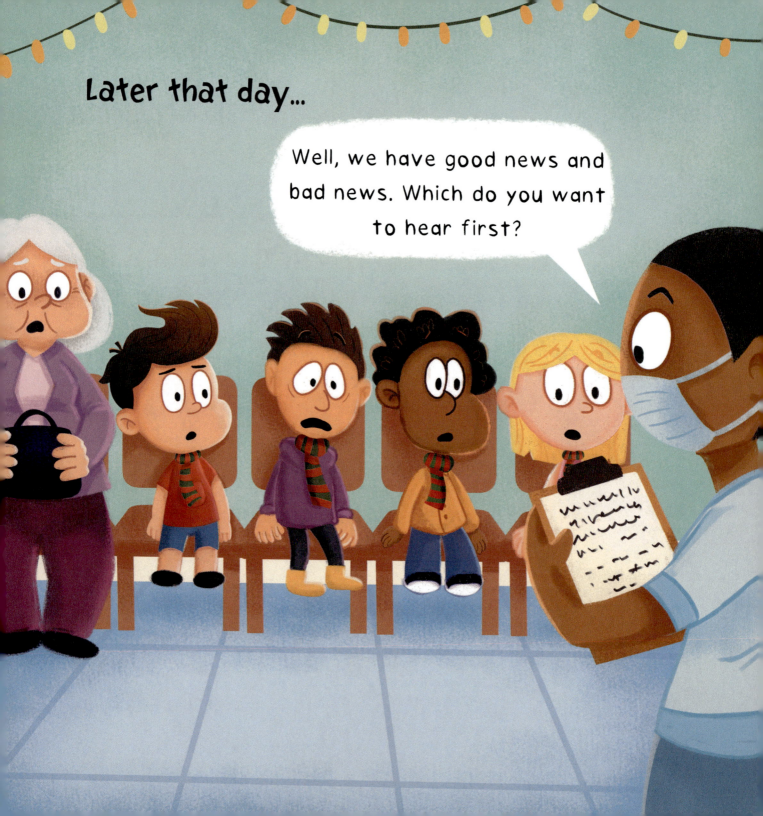

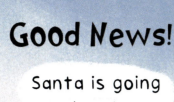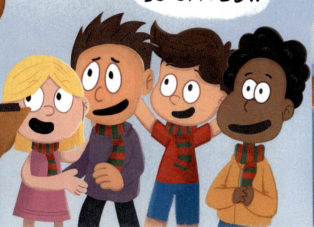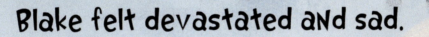

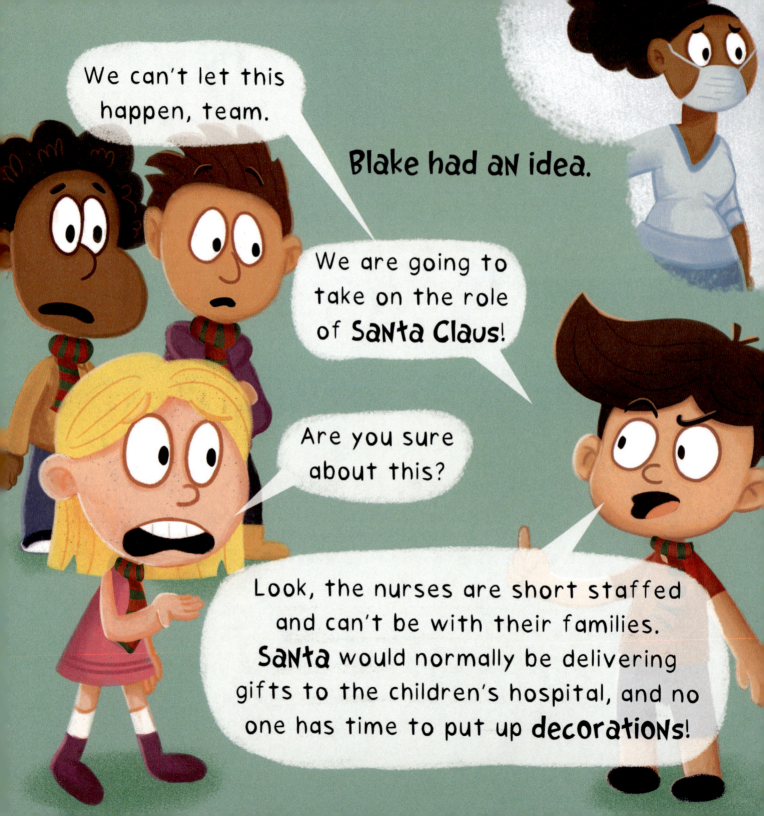

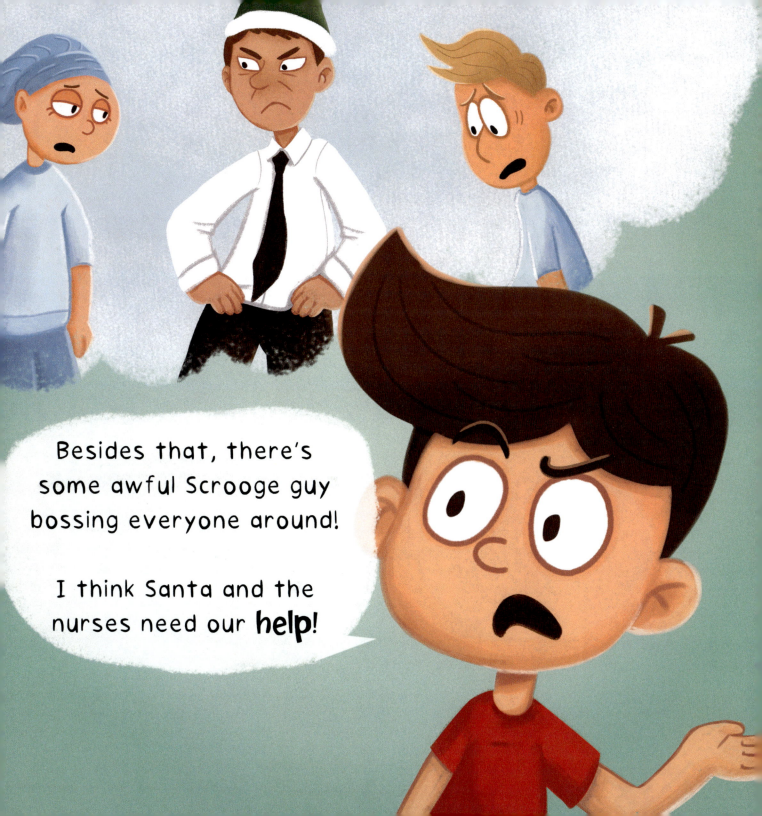

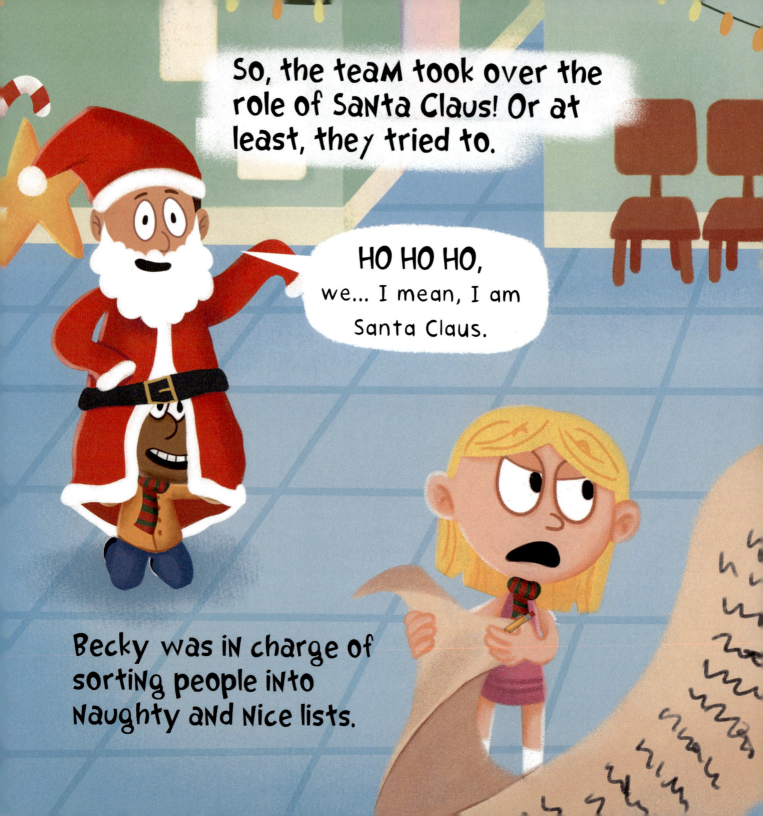

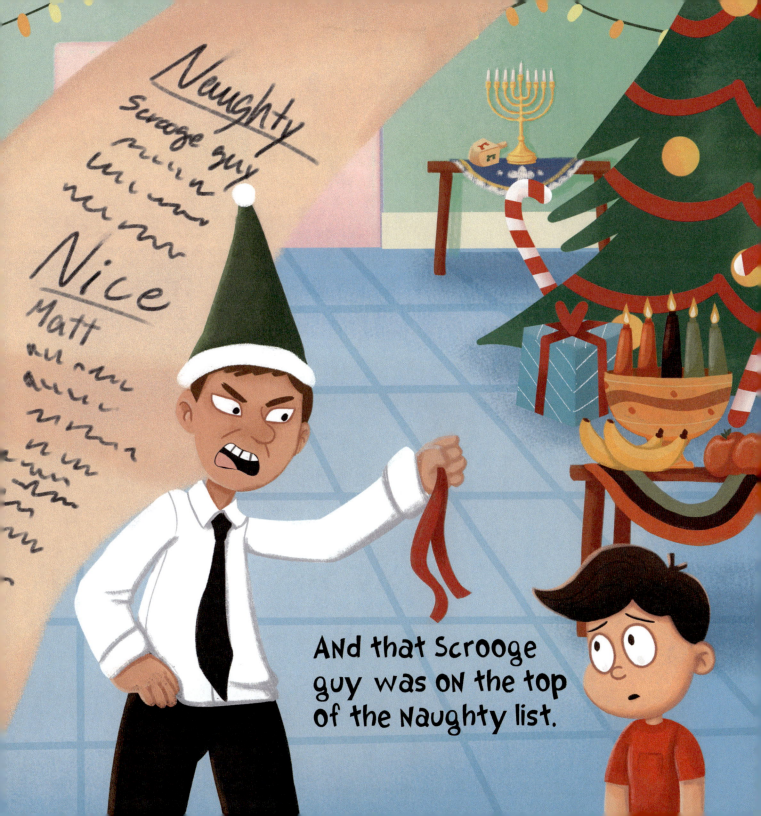

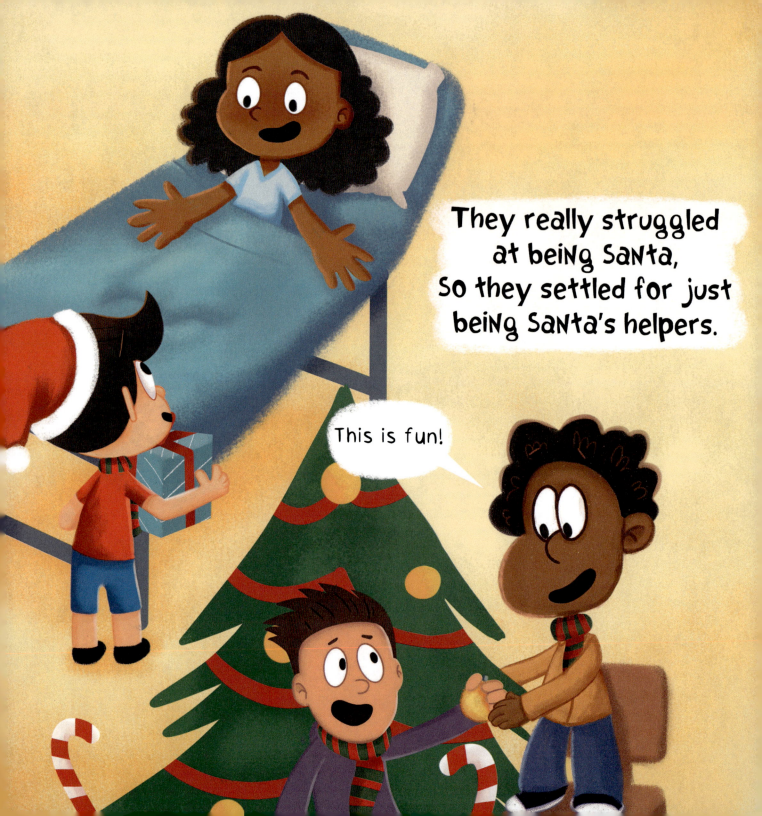

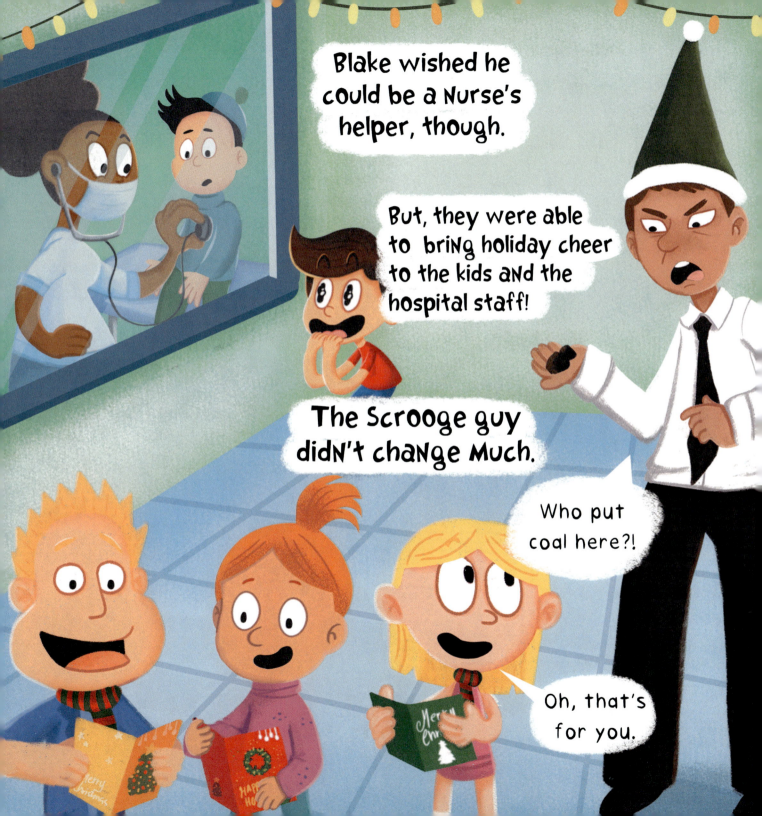

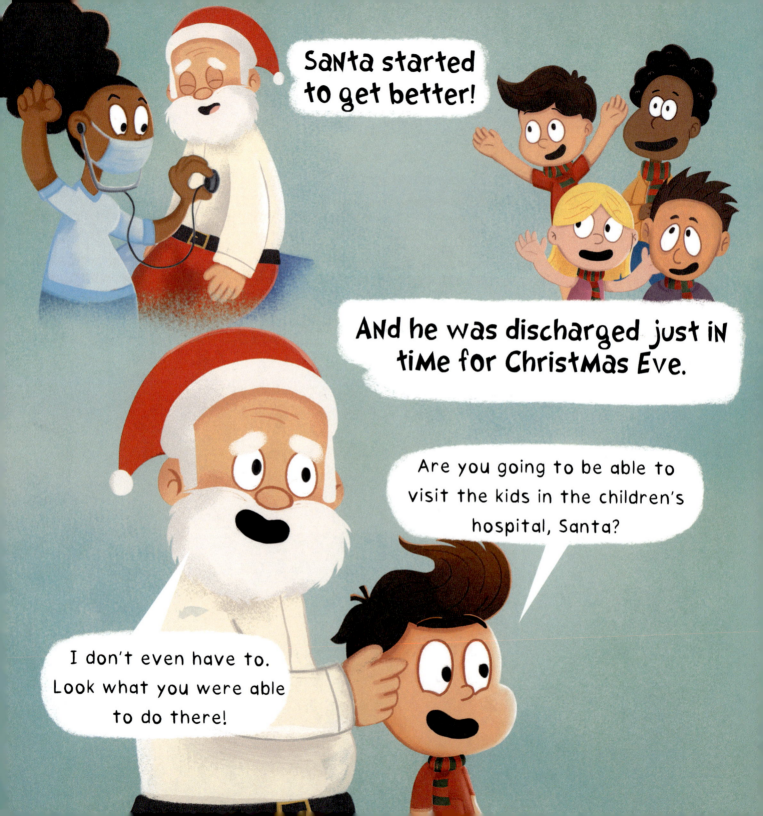

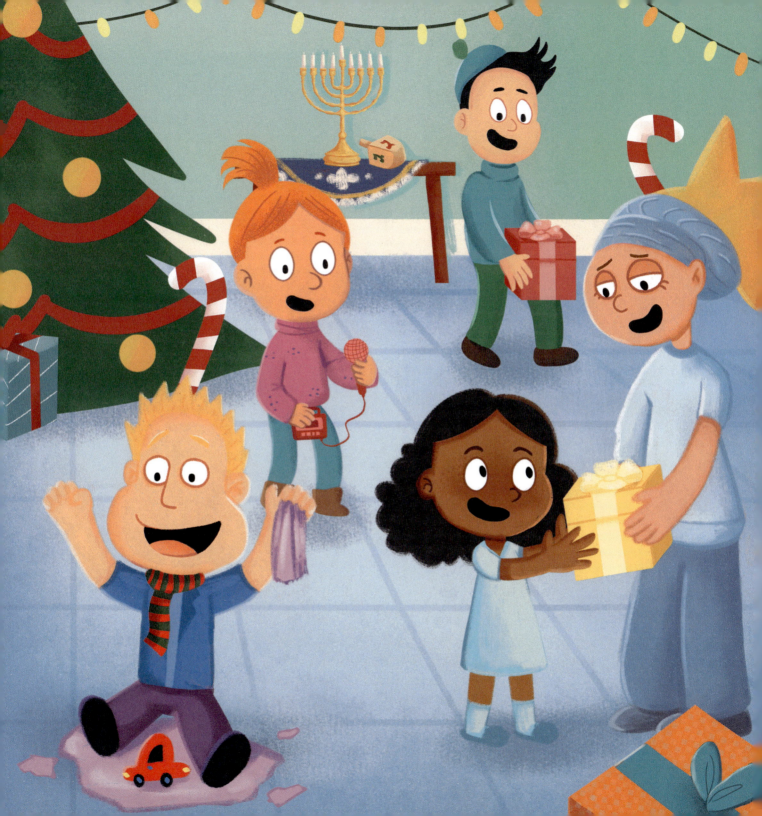

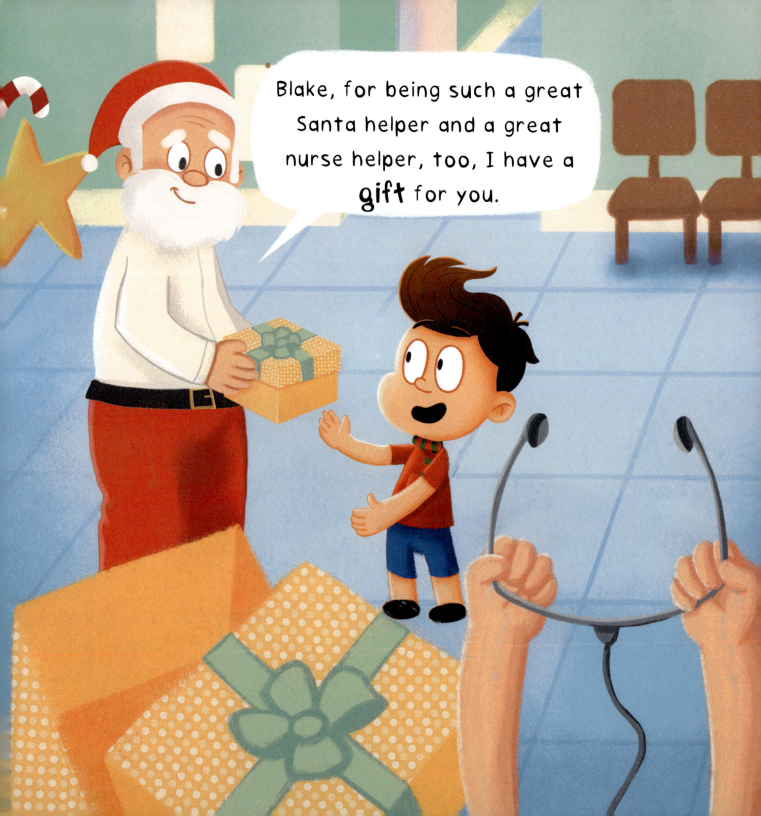

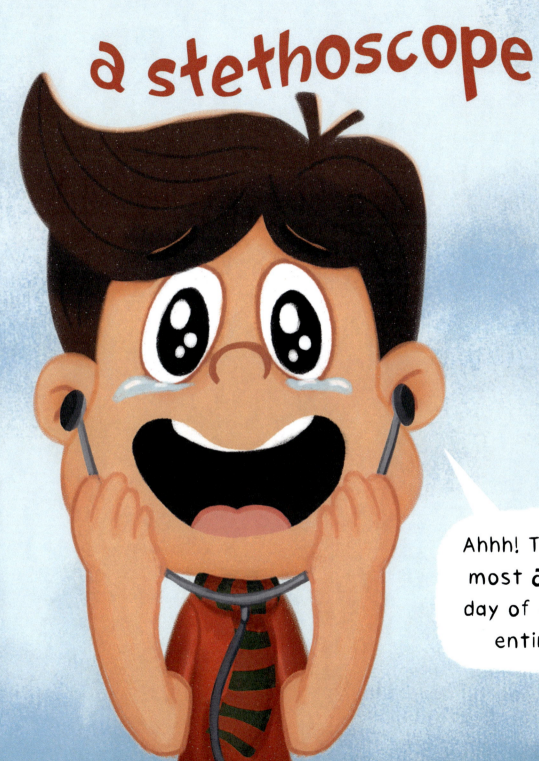

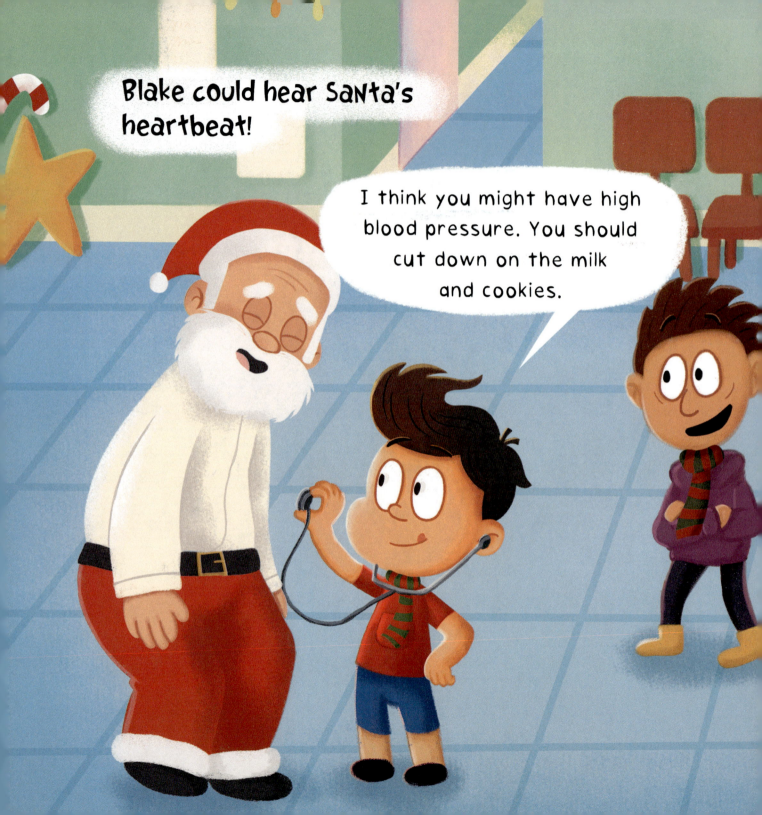

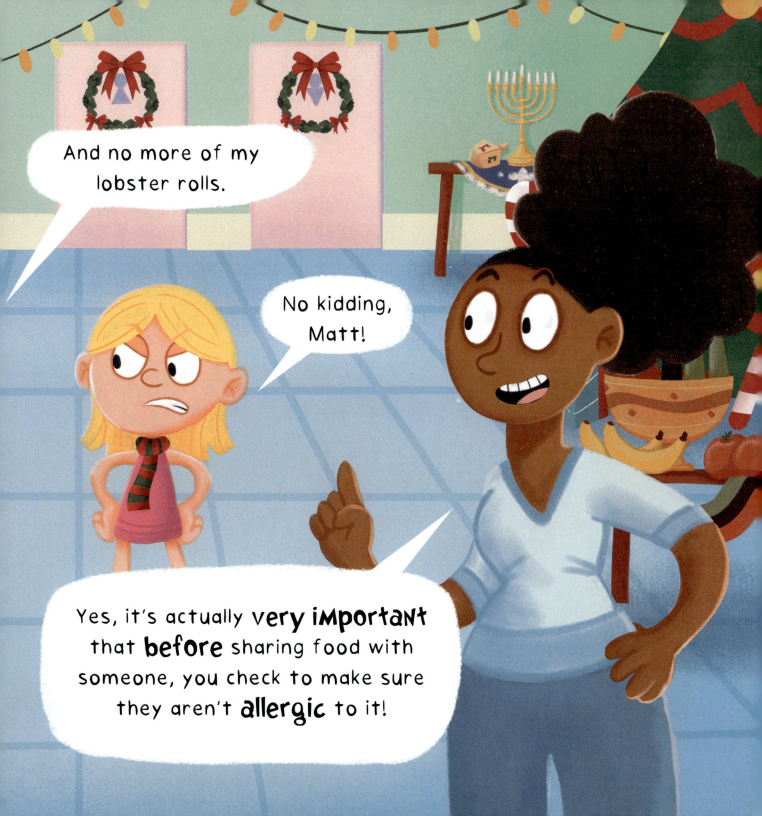

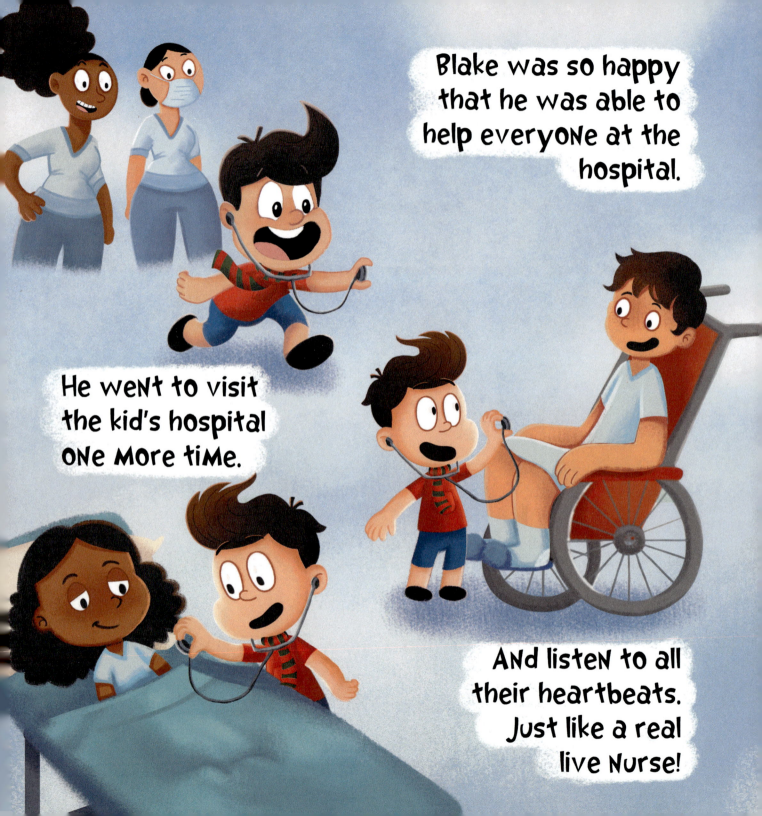

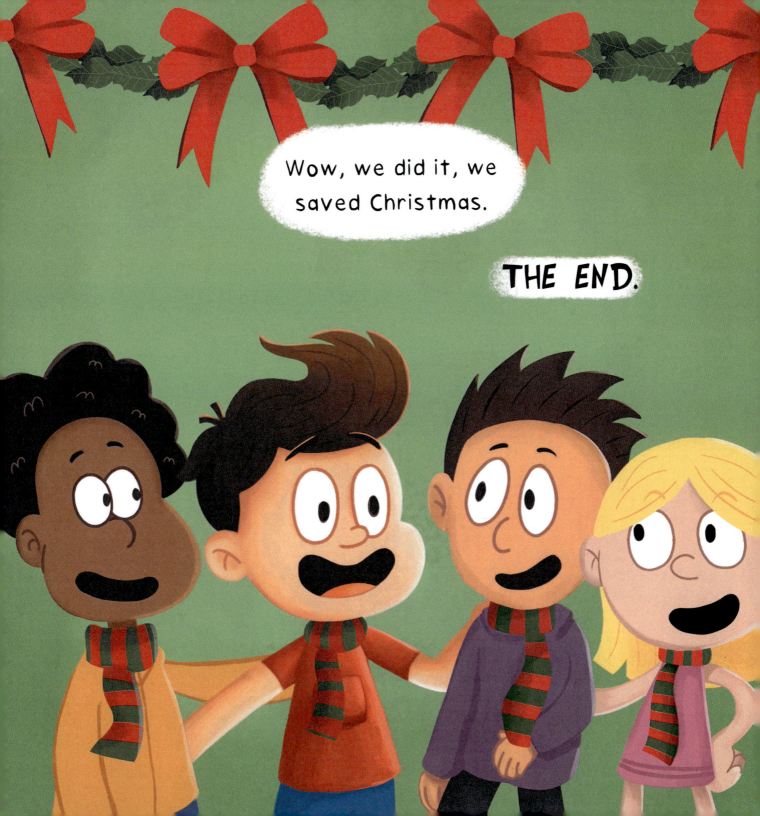

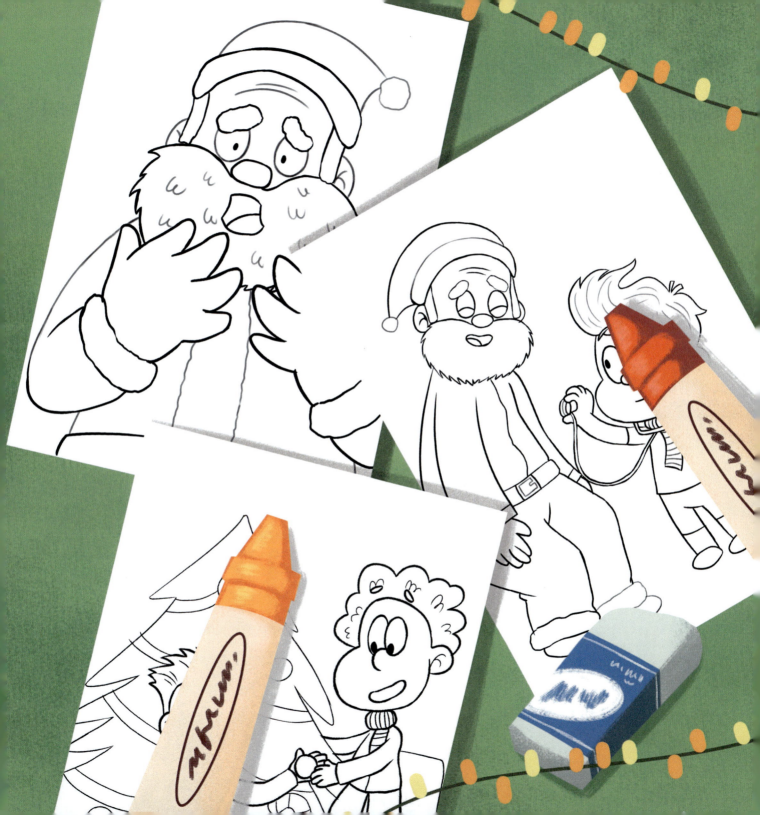

Made in the USA
Las Vegas, NV
17 October 2023

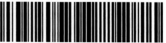

79245187R00029